SOMATIC EXERCISES FOR BEGINNERS

GLORIA CLARK

Somatic Exercises for Beginners

© 2024 by **Gloria Clark**

CONTENTS

ABOUT THE AUTHOR

Gloria Clark is an esteemed expert in the field of somatic exercises, with over two decades of experience in helping improve physical and mental well-being through mindful movement practices. As a certified expert in somatic exercises and yoga instructor, Gloria has dedicated her life to empowering others to discover the transformative power of Somatic and unlock their body's innate ability to heal and thrive.

Her journey into the world of somatic exercises began shortly after a life-changing experience that led her to explore alternative approaches to health and wellness. She had struggled with chronic pain and stress-related symptoms and had found herself on a quest to find relief and regain control over her body and mind. However, soon, she realized that traditional medical treatments offered temporary solutions but failed to address the root cause of her issues.

During this challenging time, Gloria came across a video online about somatic exercises and their profound impact on our physical and emotional well-being. Through gentle movements, breathing techniques, and mindful awareness, she began to release tension, reduce pain, and restore balance to her body. Each somatic exercise became a journey of self-discovery, allowing Gloria to reconnect with her body's wisdom and cultivate a deeper sense of presence and inner peace.

Inspired by her own transformation, Gloria decided to further continue on a path of learning and exploration, studying various somatic modalities and ancient healing practices from around the world. She became certified as a somatic exercise coach and yoga instructor, blending her anatomy, physiology, and mindfulness knowledge to create holistic programs tailored to her clients' needs due to her unique approach to somatic exercises that emphasize gentle movement, breathing awareness, and compassionate self-inquiry. Her teachings focus on relieving physical discomfort, fostering a deeper connection with oneself, and cultivating a sense of wholeness and vitality from within.

Today, Gloria is a respected authority in the field of somatic exercises, leading workshops, retreats, and teacher training programs worldwide. Her passion for helping others rediscover their innate capacity for healing and self-transformation continues to inspire countless you on their journey to health and well-being. Through her work, Clark seeks to empower others to embrace the wisdom of their bodies, reclaim their vitality, and live life to the fullest. She believes that by cultivating awareness, compassion, and resilience, anyone can overcome obstacles and thrive in mind, body, and spirit.

INTRODUCTION

Dear reader, welcome to the captivating world of somatic healing, where you can explore the incredible powers of transformation and healing. Amidst our busy and demanding lives, it is easy for us to forget to take care of ourselves and our bodies. Somatic healing offers a way for us to reconnect with our bodies and cultivate a deeper sense of well-being. This E-book serves as a manual to help you unlock the wisdom that is engraved within your bodies. Somatic exercises explained in the following chapter will guide you in enhancing your self-awareness and overall well-being instead of just simple physical exercises.

These exercises are simple body movements that involve gentle touches on the skin, which can help release the built-up tension and stiffness in your body. By paying attention to our breathing and practicing these exercises regularly, we can become more aware of our bodies and feel more comfortable and at ease in our skin. The concept behind these exercises is that our bodies act as a storage for memories, traumas, and feelings. These can cause your body to show some physical symptoms such as discomfort, tension, or even restricted bodily movements that we constantly ignore. However, you can reclaim your body's natural state of balance, health, and flexibility through somatic exercises that will unlock the stored experiences within your body. Compared to your regular workout, which includes Pilates and weightlifting, somatic-based exercises help you release stress and enhance the connection between your mind and your body. Through these exercises, we can help our brain respond to stress in healthier ways, which can help our body heal properly from the physiological effects caused by the traumas. Constant stored-up stress can trigger our bodies' natural fight or flight reaction.

In this enlightening book, *"Somatic Exercises for Beginners,"* you will learn how to tune in to your body's signals and understand what it needs. You will discover how to move in ways that feel good, breathe in a way that calms your mind, and let go of the stress and tension you may be holding onto without even realizing it. You will also learn about the science behind somatic healing and how it can help you reduce pain, improve your posture, and enhance your overall well-being. The book will guide you through a variety of exercises, from gentle stretches to more dynamic movements, so that you can find the ones that work best for you.

In this book, you will learn about the basics of somatic exercises, their benefits, foundational principles, and a personally curated list of somatic exercises, along with illustrations that will help you stay connected with your body and its reactions. It is designed to help you walk through the different facets of bodily exercises. Each chapter is curated to give you elaborated information and resources to help you achieve a fruitful somatic journey, from understanding the fundamentals of somatic exercises to addressing particular needs such as how to reduce anxiety, recover from a traumatic experience, and improve overall body posture. As you work through this book, keep in mind that somatic exercises are a means of communication with your inner self; they are not merely exercises for physical enhancement. Keep an open mind as you walk through this wonderful guide towards a life full of healing and possibilities; don't forget to leave a positive review for those in need of encouragement and help this book reach the right audience. So, get ready to discover this magical journey of somatic healing - as it awaits you to uncover its secret treasures!

Somatic Exercises for Beginners

Gloria Clark

Chapter

1

UNDERSTANDING SOMATIC

In this chapter, we will explore the fundamental principles and key concepts of somatic - a comprehensive approach to self-awareness and healing that acknowledges the interconnectedness of the mind, body, and spirit. Through introspection and investigation, we will uncover the basic principles that form the basis of somatic practice.

What is Somatic?

Somatic is an approach to movement and embodiment that is rooted in the Greek word "soma," meaning "the living body." This approach emphasizes the integration of body, mind, and spirit through an experiential process. Essentially, somatic recognizes that our physical experiences, emotions, and thought patterns are deeply interconnected and seeks to facilitate greater awareness and harmony within the whole being. By focusing on the interrelatedness of these elements, somatic allows you to develop a more profound understanding of themselves and their bodies. Through somatic practices, you can learn to move with greater ease and grace, release stored tension and trauma, and cultivate a deeper sense of inner peace and well-being.

Benefits of Somatic Exercises

Somatic exercises offer countless benefits, including enhancing your overall physical and mental well-being. These exercises provide a holistic approach to healing and self-awareness, helping you to achieve greater harmony and balance within your body-mind system. These include mindful breathing, gentle body movements, and environmental awareness, which works greatly to help release tension, increase your overall mobility, and promote a sense of complete relaxation. By engaging in somatic exercises, you can improve their overall quality of life and increase their physical and mental resilience. Whether you are looking to reduce stress, improve your posture, or simply enhance your overall well-being, somatic can be an excellent choice.

1. **Reduce Stress:** Somatic exercises enhance your body's relaxation and reduce the level of stress by activating the body's relaxin hormones and calming your nervous system. Encouraging your body to release tension and enhance your natural state of ease and relaxation helps alleviate the physical and emotional effects of stress, promoting your overall well-being and resilience.

2. **Improved Mobility and Flexibility:** Somatic exercises focus on releasing tightness and restrictions in the muscles and joints, promoting greater mobility and flexibility throughout the body. By gently stretching and mobilizing the tissues, somatic help improves the range of motion and reduce stiffness, enhancing overall movement efficiency and function.

3. **Pain Relief:** Through regular use of somatic exercising, many people have found relief from painful chronic conditions such as neck, back, and joint pain. By addressing underlying muscular tension and imbalances, somatic help alleviates pain and discomfort, allowing for greater comfort and ease in daily life.

4. **Enhanced Body Awareness:** These exercises help promote body awareness and the sense of how our bodies are positioned in the natural state. By tuning into the sensations and movements of the body with mindful awareness, you can develop a deeper understanding of their physical patterns and habits, empowering them to make positive changes and prevent injuries.

5. **Stress Reduction:** Somatic exercises promote relaxation and stress reduction by activating the body's relaxation response and calming the nervous system. By releasing tension and encouraging a state of ease and relaxation, somatic helps alleviate stress's physical and emotional effects, promoting overall well-being and resilience.

6. **Improved Posture and Alignment:** With the help of regular somatic practice, you can enhance your body's posture and alignment by releasing muscle tension and restoring overall body balance. Addressing underlying imbalances and misalignments, somatic help promote optimal biomechanics and reduce the risk of injury and strain.

How Somatic Works

Somatic is a type of therapy that is aimed to promote better self-awareness and build your overall body-mind connection. It involves gentle movement, breath work, and mindful awareness to help you tune into your body's sensations and feedback signals. This practice facilitates relaxation, release, and integration, allowing you to release tension, improve mobility, and cultivate greater well-being. The core of somatic lies in recognizing the interconnectedness of mind, body, and spirit and the profound impact our thoughts, emotions, and beliefs can have on our physical experiences. By creating awareness of this mind-body connection, somatic empowers you to explore and transform how they inhabit and experience their bodies. This promotes greater harmony, vitality, and resilience.

Through regular practice and mindful living, you can harness the transformative power of somatic to enhance their quality of life and foster a greater sense of wholeness and vitality. In essence, somatic offers a pathway to deeper self-understanding, embodied presence, and holistic well-being. It is a valuable tool for anyone seeking to release habitual patterns and embody their fullest potential.

2

FOUNDATIONAL PRINCIPLES OF SOMATIC EXERCISES

In this chapter, we will explore the foundational principles underpinning somatic exercises, focusing on developing body awareness, cultivating mindful attention to body sensations, and recognizing tension patterns within the body.

Body Awareness

Body awareness lies at the heart of somatic practice, encompassing the ability to tune into the sensations, movements, and feedback signals of the body with mindful attention. Developing body awareness involves cultivating a deep connection with the physical body, exploring its nuances and subtleties, and honoring its inherent wisdom. Through somatic exercises, you learn to listen to the body's language, recognize its messages, and respond with care and compassion.

Developing Awareness of Body Sensations

Central to somatic practice is the cultivation of awareness of body sensations – the felt experiences of the body in the present moment. By tuning into sensations such as warmth, tension, relaxation, and movement, you can deepen their understanding of their bodies and gain insight into their physical and emotional states. Through gentle movement, breath work, and mindful attention, you learn to navigate the landscape of their bodies with curiosity and openness, fostering greater self-awareness and self-compassion.

Recognizing Tension Patterns

One of the critical aims of somatic exercises is to identify and release tension patterns within the body. Tension patterns often manifest as tightness, stiffness, or discomfort resulting from habitual movement patterns, emotional stress, or past injuries. Through somatic practice, you learn to identify these tension patterns through mindful attention and observation, bringing awareness to areas of tightness and restriction. By recognizing tension patterns, you can unravel and release chronic muscular holding, promoting relaxation and ease within the body.

Integration and Embodiment

Ultimately, the goal of somatic practice is to integrate body, mind, and spirit, fostering a deep sense of embodiment and wholeness. By cultivating body awareness, mindful attention to sensations, and recognition of tension patterns, you can align yourself with your body's innate intelligence, promoting greater harmony, vitality, and well-being. By honoring the interconnectedness of body, mind, and spirit, somatic empowers you to inhabit their bodies with presence, grace, and authenticity, fostering a deeper connection with themselves and the world around them.

In other words, the foundational principles of somatic exercises center on the development of body awareness, the development of mindful attention to body sensations, and the recognition of tension patterns within the body. By following these principles, you can start on a journey of self-discovery and transformation, tapping into the inherent wisdom of your body and fostering greater well-being and vitality.

3

BREATH AND RELAXATION IN SOMATIC PRACTICE

In this chapter, we will explore the integral role that breath and relaxation play in somatic practice. We'll delve into the relationship between breath and bodily tension and examine how conscious breathing techniques can promote relaxation, release tension, and enhance overall well-being.

The Importance of Breath

Breath serves as a bridge between the mind and body, influencing your physiological state and emotional well-being. In somatic practice, conscious breathing is a powerful tool for promoting relaxation, reducing stress, and fostering greater body awareness. By focusing on the quality and rhythm of your breathing, you can connect deeply with your body and encourage a better sense of calm.

Deep Breathing Technique for Stress Relief

It is a simple and powerful technique used to help promote relaxation, reduce stress, and enhance your overall well-being. By engaging the diaphragm and taking slow, deep breaths, you can activate the body's relaxation response, calm the nervous system, and promote a sense of calm and tranquility. Here are a few ways you can use this technique for stress relief:

1. *Find a Suitable Position:* Begin by sitting or standing in a position you are comfortable with, and keep your spine aligned and shoulders relaxed.

2. *Close your eyes:* Close your eyes and divert your attention to yourself and your whole body.

3. *Inhale deeply:* Start taking a slow and deep breath inside using your nostrils, and fill your lungs with as much air as you can.

4. *Exhale slowly:* Then, exhale the air slowly and thoroughly through your mouth, relaxing your tummy as you breathe.

5. *Repeat:* Continue breathing in and out slowly and focus on the sensation of your breath moving in and out of your body. Allow each breath to be smooth, steady, and relaxed.

6. *Set a rhythm:* Establishing a rhythm for your breath is helpful as you practice deep breathing. For example, you can set a specific number for each inhale and exhale, so inhale and count, then exhale and count. Experiment with different rhythms to find what feels most comfortable for you.

7. *Practice regularly:* Set aside a few minutes each day to practice deep breathing for stress relief. You can incorporate deep breathing into your morning routine, take a few moments to practice during a break at work, or use it as a relaxation technique before bedtime.

Breathe work for Stress Relief

In addition to deep breathing, several breath work techniques can be used to promote stress relief and relaxation. Here are a few examples:

1. **4-7-8 Breathing:** Inhale for a count of four, hold your breath for a count of seven, and exhale for eight. This technique is used to help enhance your body's reaction and improve your sense of calmness.

2. **Alternate Nostril Breathing:** Use your thumb to close one nostril and breathe in deeply through the open nostril. Then, repeat the same on the other nostril with

your ring finger and breathe out through the first nostril. Continue to switch between both your nostrils with each breath. This technique can help balance the flow of energy in the body and promote a sense of calm.

3. **Equal Breathing:** Breathe in and out for an equal count, such as inhaling for a count of 5 and exhaling for a count of 5. This technique can help promote balance and stability in the mind and body.

4. **Breathe Counting:** Count the number of breaths you take, starting from one and going up to ten. Include both inhalation and exhalation in your counting. Then, start again at one. If you lose count, simply start over. This technique can help quiet the mind and promote focus and concentration.

Experiment with these different breathwork techniques to find what works best for you. Incorporate them into your daily routine as a tool for stress relief, relaxation, and overall well-being. By including mindful breathing techniques in your regular exercise practice, you can use your breath to enhance greater calm, resilience, and peace of mind.

4

MOVEMENT EXPLORATIONS IN SOMATIC PRACTICE

This chapter will delve into the rich and varied landscape of movement explorations within somatic practice. We will explore how movement can be used as a vehicle for self-discovery, healing, and transformation. We will learn about various somatic movement techniques designed to promote awareness, release tension, and enhance well-being.

Gentle Movement Sequences and Exploring Range of Motion

In somatic practice, gentle movement sequences are crucial in promoting body awareness, releasing tension, and enhancing overall well-being. These sequences are designed to be slow, deliberate, and mindful, allowing you to explore their range of motion with curiosity and compassion. Here is how gentle movement sequences and exploring the range of motion can benefit somatic practice:

1. **Gentle Movement Sequences:** Gentle movement sequences in somatic practice involve a series of slow, flowing movements designed to promote relaxation, release tension, and improve mobility. These sequences may include movements such as:

   (a) *Slow Spinal Rolls:* Slowly rolling the spine allows the body to release tension and find ease in movement.

(b) *Shoulder Circles:* Circling the shoulders in a slow, controlled manner to release tension in the neck and shoulders and improve shoulder mobility.

(c) *Hip Circles:* Gently rotating the hips in circular motions to release tension in the hip joints and promote hip mobility.

(d) *Cat-Cow Stretches:* Moving between a rounded spine (cat) and an arched spine (cow) to release tension in the spine and promote spinal flexibility.

2. **Exploring Range of Motion:** Exploring range of motion in somatic practice involves gradually moving the body through its full range of motion with awareness and intention. This allows you to identify areas of tightness or restriction and gently explore ways to release tension and improve mobility. Some techniques for exploring range of motion include:

(a) *Joint Mobilization Exercises:* Gently moving the joints through their full range of motion to smoothen them, improve joint mobility, and reduce stiffness.

(b) *Active Stretching:* Engaging specific muscle groups to actively stretch and lengthen them, promoting flexibility and releasing tension.

(c) *Slow, Mindful Movement:* Moving slowly and deliberately through a series of movements, paying close attention to the sensations and feedback signals of your body.

Benefits of Gentle Movement Sequences and Exploring Range of Motion

1. *Promotes Body Awareness:* Gentle movement sequences and exploring the range of motion help you tune into the sensations of their bodies, enhancing their sense of awareness and presence.

2. *Releases Tension:* By moving slowly and mindfully, you can identify areas of tension and explore ways to release it, promoting relaxation and reducing muscular holding patterns.

3. *Improves Mobility:* Gentle movement sequences and exploring range of motion help improve joint mobility and flexibility, allowing you to move more freely and with greater ease.

4. *Enhances Overall Well-Being:* Engaging in gentle movement sequences and exploring range of motion can have a profound impact on overall well-being, promoting relaxation, reducing stress, and enhancing physical and mental resilience.

In conclusion, gentle movement sequences and exploring range of motion are essential components of somatic practice, offering a pathway to greater body awareness, relaxation, and mobility. By incorporating these practices into their daily routine, you can create a deeper connection with their bodies and experience greater ease and vitality.

Chapter

5

UPPER BODY SOMATIC EXERCISES

Somatic exercises are focused on increasing awareness and sensations of your body whilst putting your body in relaxation mode and ease of movement. In comparison to the traditional workouts that include painful stretching or heavy weight lifting, somatic exercises promote mindful bodily movements and breathing techniques to release any built-up tension and improve not only your physical body but also your overall well-being.

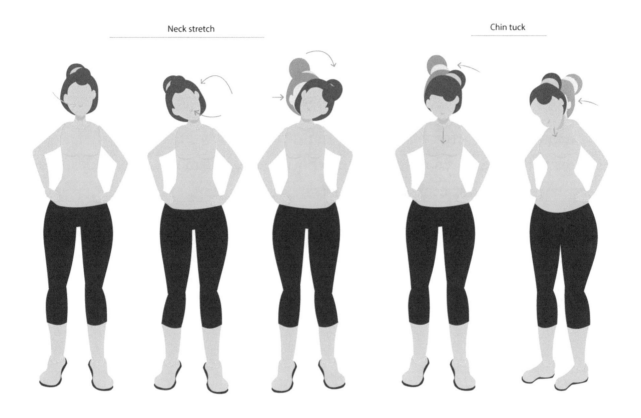

Somatic Exercise for Neck Tension Release

This exercise can help release neck tension and promote relaxation. Practicing it regularly can increase awareness of neck tension and lead to greater comfort and ease of movement.

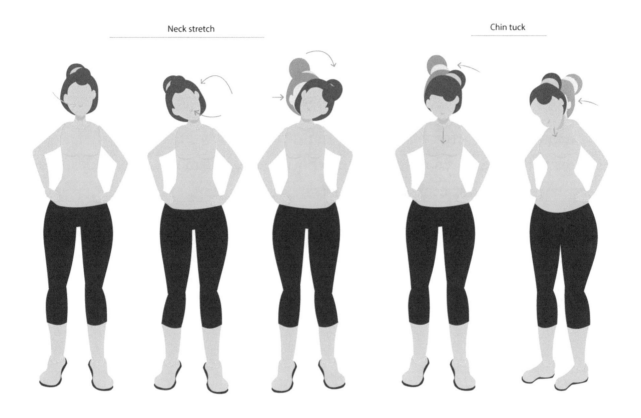

1. *Find a Suitable Position:* Begin by sitting or standing in a position you are comfortable with, and keep your spine aligned and shoulders relaxed.

2. *Deep Breathing:* Close your eyes and take a few deep breaths through your nose; feel your chest and belly expand as you inhale, and notice any tension or tightness in your neck.

3. *Stretch your Neck:* Gently tilt your head to one side, bringing your ear towards your shoulder as you breathe in. Be careful and only stretch as far as it feels comfortable; hold this position for a moment.

4. *Breathe Into the Stretch:* As you hold the stretch, take a few deep breaths, focusing on sending your breath into the tight areas of your neck. Imagine stress melting away with each breath.

5. *Switch Sides:* As you exhale, slowly return your head to the center, and then repeat the stretch on the opposite side.

6. *Chin Tuck:* After stretching both sides of your neck, bring your head back to the center. Then, repeat what you did on your sides and gently tuck your chin towards your chest. Hold this position till you feel the stretch along the back of your neck.

7. *Release and Relax:* After holding the chin tuck for a few breaths, slowly release and allow your head to return to its natural position. Take a moment to relax and notice any changes in your neck and shoulders.

8. *Roll the Shoulders:* Roll your shoulders to the front and back a few times to release the built-up tension in your upper body.

9. *Mindful Relaxation:* Take a few deep breaths in and out, relax, and release any tension in your neck. Open your eyes when you're ready.

Somatic Exercise for Shoulder Relaxation

This exercise helps release shoulder tension caused by stress, poor posture, or repetitive movements. Practicing it regularly increases awareness of shoulder tension and promotes relaxation.

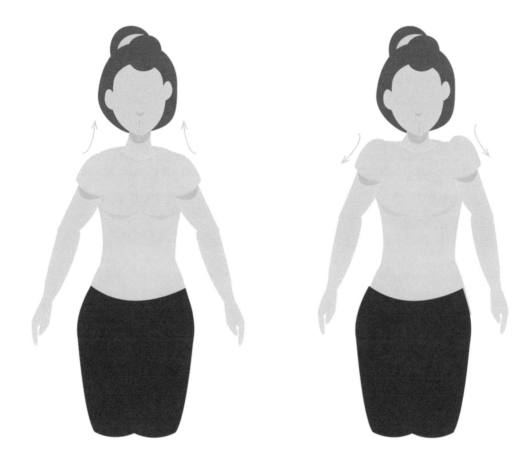

1. *Find a Comfortable Position:* Begin by finding a comfortable seated or standing position. Sit or stand tall with your spine aligned and your shoulders relaxed.

2. *Deep Breathing:* Take deep breaths through your nose and feel your chest and belly expand as you inhale. Notice any shoulder tension or tightness.

3. *Shoulder Shrugs:* Shrug your shoulders towards your ears while inhaling. Hold the position for a moment.

4. *Release on Exhale:* As you exhale, slowly release your shoulders back down, allowing them to relax and soften. Focus on letting go of any tension or tightness as you breathe out.

5. *Repeat Shoulder Shrugs:* Repeat the shoulder shrug with each inhale and release with each exhale.

6. *Shoulder Rolls:* Roll your shoulders towards your ears, then back and down in circles. Repeat this several times for a free and natural movement.

7. *Reverse Shoulder Rolls:* Reverse the direction of your shoulder rolls and repeat several times. Then, relax your shoulders and notice any sensations. Finally, take a few deep breaths and release any remaining tension.

Somatic Exercise for Upper Trapezius Stretch

This exercise targets the upper trapezius muscles, which can become tense due to stress, poor posture, or repetitive movements. Regular practice can help relieve tension and improve comfort and movement.

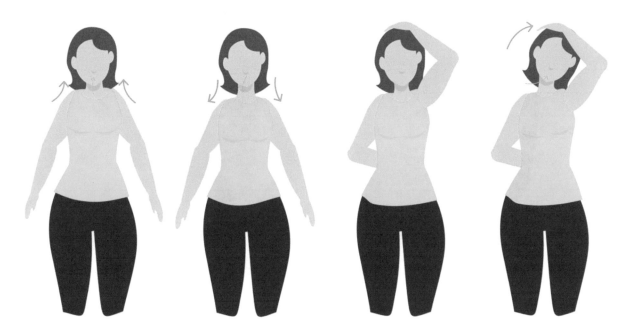

1. *Find a Comfortable Position:* Sit or stand tall with relaxed shoulders and spine aligned.

2. *Deep Breathing:* Take deep breaths through your nose and feel your chest and belly expand as you inhale. Notice any shoulder tension or tightness.

3. *Shoulder Drop:* Inhale and lift your shoulders towards your ears, feeling the stretch.

4. *Exhale and Drop:* Drop your shoulders down and away from your ears as you exhale to release tension in the upper trapezius muscles.

5. *Repeat Shoulder Drops:* Repeat the shoulder drop movement by inhaling and releasing with exhalation. Notice changes in trapezius muscle tension.

6. *Neck Tilt:* Add a neck tilt to the shoulder drop stretch. Inhale and tilt your head to one side, bringing your ear towards your shoulder while keeping both shoulders relaxed. Hold for a moment and feel the stretch along the side of your neck and upper trapezius.

7. *Breathe Into the Stretch:* Take deep breaths as you hold the stretch; imagine the tension melting away with each exhale.

8. *Switch Sides:* Tilt your head to one side, hold for a few breaths, then repeat on the other side. Be gentle and move only as far as feels comfortable.

9. *Relaxation:* Relax your shoulders and neck after stretching them. Let your shoulders rest in their natural position and notice any changes in tension.

10. *Closing Breaths:* Take a few deep breaths in and out, relax your upper trapezius muscles, and when you're ready, gently open your eyes.

Somatic Exercise for Shoulder Rolls

Shoulder rolls release tension and promote relaxation in the upper back. Practicing this exercise regularly increases awareness of tension in these areas, leading to greater comfort and ease of movement.

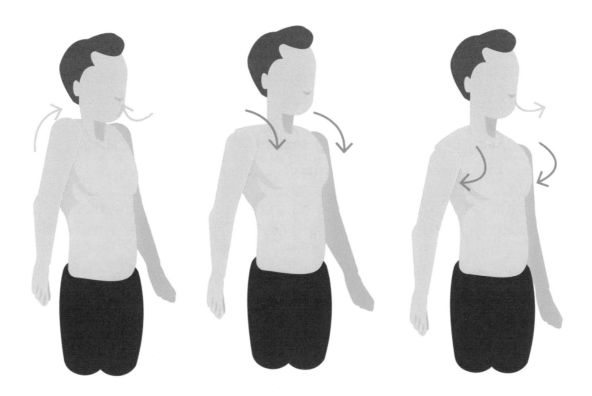

1. *Find a Comfortable Position:* Sit or stand tall with relaxed shoulders and spine aligned.

2. *Deep Breathing:* Take deep breaths through your nose and feel your chest and belly expand as you inhale. Notice any shoulder tension or tightness.

3. *Shoulder Lift:* Inhale and lift both shoulders towards your ears. Hold for a moment as you feel a stretch.

4. *Roll the Shoulders Back:* Roll both shoulders back and down in a circular motion while exhaling. Trace a circle with your shoulders towards your back and then down towards your hips.

5. *Complete the Circle:* Roll your shoulders in smooth circles with intention, completing a full rotation.

6. *Reverse the Direction:* After completing several shoulder rolls in one direction, reverse the direction of your circles.

7. *Breathe Into the Movement:* Sync your breath with your shoulder rolls. Inhale as you lift them, exhale as you roll them back and down.

8. *Mindful Relaxation:* Take a few deep breaths in and out, relax, and release any tension in your neck. Open your eyes when you're ready.

9. *Closing Breaths:* Take a few deep breaths in and out, relax your upper trapezius muscles, and when you're ready, gently open your eyes.

Somatic Exercise for Neck Circles

Neck circles are a gentle somatic exercise designed to release tension and promote relaxation in the neck and upper shoulders.

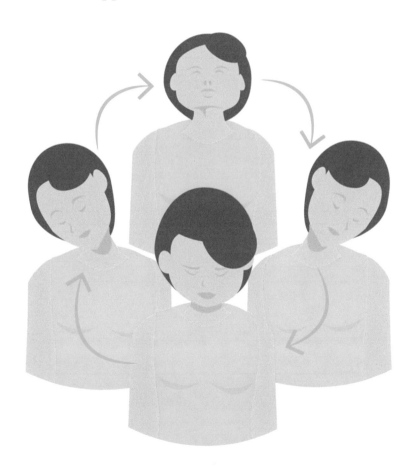

1. *Find a Comfortable Position:* Sit or stand tall with relaxed shoulders and spine aligned.

2. *Deep Breathing:* Take deep breaths through your nose and feel your chest and belly expand as you inhale. Notice any shoulder tension or tightness.

3. *Neck Rotation:* Tilt your head to one side while inhaling and bring your ear towards your shoulder. Hold for a moment and feel the stretch on the side of your neck.

4. *Circle Motion:* Gently roll your head in a circular motion, tracing a circle with your nose. Move from chin to chest, over to the opposite shoulder, and back to the starting position.

5. *Reverse Direction:* After completing several neck circles in one direction, reverse the direction of your circles.

6. *Breathe Into the Movement:* Sync your breath with head circles. Inhale as you begin, exhale as you complete. This helps ease tension in the neck and shoulders.

7. *Mindful Relaxation:* After doing neck circles, relax your neck and shoulders. Observe any changes in tension or relaxation.

8. *Closing Breaths:* Take a few deep breaths in and out, relax your upper trapezius muscles, and when you're ready, gently open your eyes.

Chapter

6

SOMATIC EXERCISES FOR SPINAL MOBILITY

In this chapter, we'll explore somatic exercises to improve spinal mobility, flexibility, and overall health. Maintaining mobility in the spine is crucial for promoting proper posture, reducing injury risk, and enhancing overall well-being. Poor posture, sedentary lifestyle habits, and aging can contribute to stiffness and decreased mobility in the spine, but targeted exercises can help restore and maintain spinal mobility, leading to improved posture, reduced pain, and enhanced quality of life.

Somatic Exercise: Cat-Cow Stretch

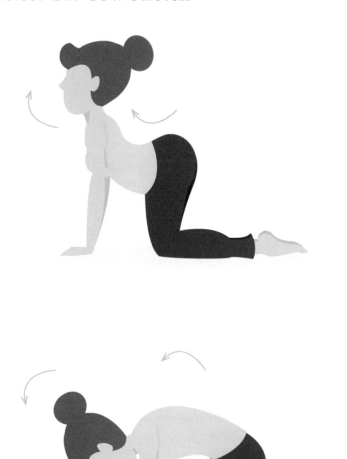

It is one of the foundational exercises included in every somatic routine that helps enhance the flexibility, mobility, and overall posture of your spine. It includes alternating movements between arching and rounding the back. It is beneficial for relieving tension in the spine, promoting relaxation, and enhancing body awareness.

1. *Starting Position:* Start in a tabletop position with wrists under shoulders and knees under hips. Keep the spine in a natural state with a slight curve in your lower back.

2. *Inhale in Cow Position:* Move your lower back in an arch position by dropping your belly and lifting your head and chest upwards. Squeeze the space between blades in

your shoulder and open up the front of your body. Keep your gaze forward or slightly upward based on your comfort level.

3. *Exhale in Cat Position:* Move your pelvis under by rounding your spine, and bring your chin towards your chest as you breathe. Engage your abs and push into your hands and knees, stretching your spine. Let your head tilt towards the floor.

4. *Flowing Movement:* Transition smoothly between Cow and Cat positions, syncing breath with movement. Inhale, belly drops, chest lifts for Cow. Exhale, round spine, draw belly in for Cat. Move at your pace; let breath guide you.

5. *Repeat:* Continue to repeat for at least 5-10 rounds as a part of your routine. At least 2 sets of 5 rounds each can be added to your warm-up or cool-down routines.

Somatic Exercise: Pelvic Tilts Used for Spine Alignment

This exercise is one of the basic somatic exercises used to improve the functionality and flexibility of your lower back, abdomen, and pelvis.

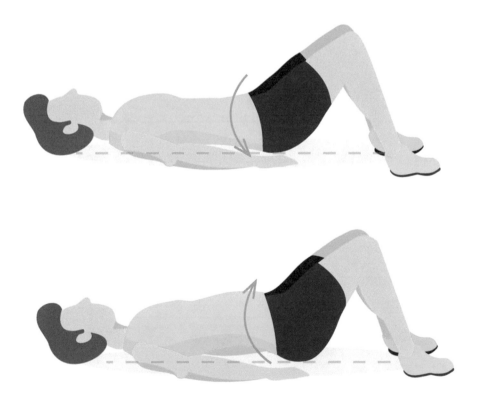

1. *Starting Position:* Start by comfortably lying down on the ground with your knees bent and feet flat on the ground. Keep arms by your sides with palms facing down.

2. *Neutral Spine:* Align your spine by pressing your lower back into the floor and lengthening your tailbone towards your heels.

3. *Engage Abdominal Muscles:* Exhale and engage your abs by pulling your navel towards your spine. This stabilizes your pelvis and preps your core for pelvic tilt.

4. *Pelvic Tilt:* Inhale and prepare. Exhale, push your lower back against the floor by tilting your pelvis towards your belly button. Feel your abdominal muscles engage and allow your tailbone to lift slightly.

5. *Hold and Release:* Hold the pelvic tilt position for a few seconds, engaging your abs and keeping your breath steady. Inhale to release and feel the natural curve returning to your lower back. Repeat exhaling to tilt, flatten, and inhale to release and arch your lower back.

6. *Flowing Movement:* Transition smoothly between pelvic tilt and release, syncing your breath with movement.

7. *Mindful Awareness:* Feel the sensations in the lower back, abdomen, and pelvis during pelvic tilts. Adjust the tilt intensity based on any tension or restriction felt. Mindfully observe the impact on overall posture.

8. *Repetition and Duration:* Aim to repeat this at least 10-15 reps, gradually increasing the number once you become comfortable with it. Adding it to your everyday routine will help maintain spine alignment and support overall spinal health.

Somatic Exercise: Seated Spinal Twist

This exercise is used to improve mobility, release tension in back muscles, and promote overall flexibility of your spine. It targets muscles along the spine, shoulders, and hips, helping to alleviate stiffness and discomfort.

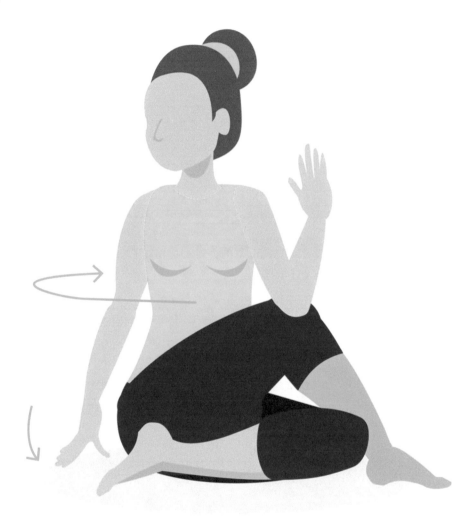

1. *Starting Position:* Sit on the floor with legs extended in front. Keep your spine straight and shoulders relaxed. Stretch arms out to sides at shoulder height, palms facing down.

2. *Bend the Right Knee:* Put your right leg crossing over your left leg and place it on the floor near your left thigh.

3. *Inhale to Lengthen:* Take a deep breath and lift your chest slightly to gently stretch your torso.

4. *Exhale to Twist:* Exhale, engage the core, and rotate the torso to the right from the spine base. Place left hand on the outside of right knee for guidance. Keep your right hand on the floor behind your hip for support.

5. *Lengthen with Each Inhale:* As you exhale, stretch your spine upward, as if you are adding space along your entire spinal length.

6. *Deepen the Twist with Each Exhale:* Slowly and mindfully twist your core muscles slightly more to your right with each exhale.

7. *Gaze Over the Right Shoulder:* Follow your gaze along with the twist, keeping your neck relaxed and chin aligned with the floor in a comfortable and natural position.

8. *Hold and Breathe:* Keep your spinal twist for 3-5 breaths and maintain a steady and even breathing pattern throughout.

9. *Release the Twist:* Slowly release the twist by unwinding from the pose and returning to your natural spinal state.

10. *Repeat on the Other Side:* Now, repeat the same twist using your left side and follow the same steps in the opposite direction. Continue this for 5-10 reps on each side.

Somatic Exercise: Sphinx Pose

Sphinx Pose is a gentle somatic exercise that helps improve spinal flexibility, alleviate lower back discomfort, and promote relaxation. It targets the muscles along the spine, particularly the erector spinal muscles, while gently stretching the chest, abdomen, and shoulders.

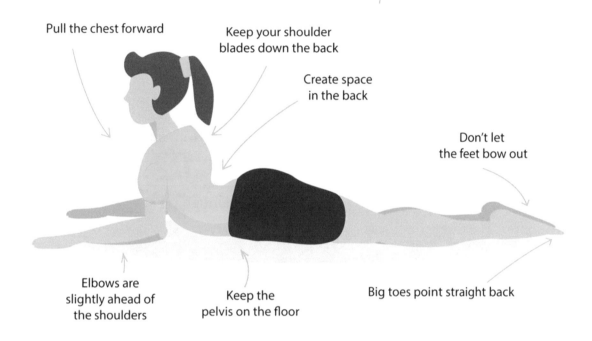

Pull the chest forward

Keep your shoulder blades down the back

Create space in the back

Don't let the feet bow out

Elbows are slightly ahead of the shoulders

Keep the pelvis on the floor

Big toes point straight back

1. *Starting Position:* Lie on your stomach with your legs extended and the top of your feet on the floor. Place your forehead gently on the mat and extend your arms relaxed alongside your body.

2. *Position Your Elbows:* Place your forearms on the floor parallel to each other and shoulder-width apart, ensuring they are positioned close to your torso.

3. *Engage Your Core:* Engage your stomach muscles by drawing your belly towards your spine.

4. *Press into Your Forearms:* Press your forearms firmly while lifting your chest and upper body off the floor as you breathe.

5. *Lengthen Your Spine:* As you lift your chest, lengthen your spine by reaching the top of your head forward and lifting through your chest. Avoid collapsing into your lower back or hyperextending your neck.

6. *Open Your Chest:* Roll your shoulders back and down, gently opening your chest and drawing your shoulder blades towards each other. Keep your shoulders relaxed away from your ears.

7. *Keep Your Hips Grounded:* Ensure that your hips remain grounded on the floor throughout the pose. Avoid lifting your hips or arching your lower back excessively.

8. *Gaze Forward:* Soften your gaze and look forward, keeping your neck aligned with your spine. Avoid straining your neck by dropping your head back or looking up too high.

9. *Hold the Pose:* Hold for 30 seconds to 1 minute, maintaining steady and even breaths throughout the pose. Focus on your overall posture.

10. *Release the Pose:* To release Sphinx Pose, gently lower your chest and upper body back down to the floor, resting your forehead on the mat.

Somatic Exercise: Child's Pose

Child's Pose is a fundamental yoga pose often used for grounding and calming the mind and body.

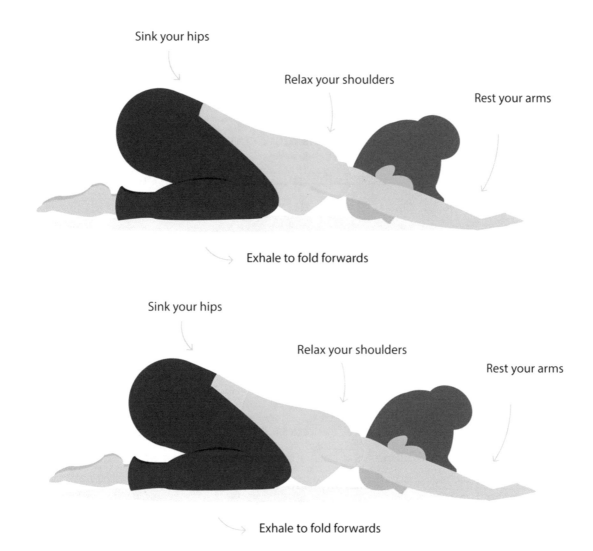

1. *Starting Position:* Start by sitting on the floor in a kneeling position with your knees apart and your big toes touching behind you. Sit on your heels and balance yourself till you are comfortable.

2. *Inhale to Lengthen:* As you breathe in, start stretching your spine upward, reaching the top of your head upwards. Feel a gentle stretch along the front of your torso.

3. *Exhale to Fold Forward:* Slowly breathe out and lower your torso forward, bending your hips, and bring your forehead towards the mat.

4. *Rest Your Arms:* Extend your arms out in front of you, palms facing down, or bring your arms alongside your body with your palms facing up.

5. *Relax Your Shoulders:* Release any tension in your shoulders and neck by allowing your arms to rest heavily on the mat. Relax your shoulders away from your ears.

6. *Sink Your Hips:* Sink your hips towards your heels, allowing your buttocks to rest on your heels or on the floor if that feels more comfortable.

7. *Breathe Deeply:* Take deep, slow breaths in and out through your nose, focusing on expanding your ribcage with each inhale and relaxing deeper into the pose with each exhale.

8. *Hold the Pose:* Hold for 1-3 minutes, or longer if desired, allowing yourself to fully surrender to the posture and the present moment. Feel the sense of relaxation with each breath.

9. *Release the Pose:* To release, slowly walk your hands back towards your body, lifting your torso back up to a seated position.

Incorporating regular spinal mobility exercises can improve posture, flexibility, and overall spinal health. These exercises promote optimal function and reduce the risk of injury and discomfort. Practice mindfully and adjust as needed for safe and effective movement. With consistency and dedication, enjoy improved spinal mobility and enhanced well-being.

7

HIP AND PELVIC STABILITY SOMATIC EXERCISES

In this chapter, we'll explore somatic exercises for hip and pelvic stability. These exercises enhance body awareness, mobility, and function. Practicing regularly can promote balance, stability, and comfort. The hips and pelvis provide support for the movement, and maintaining stability is essential for proper alignment, injury prevention, and functional movement patterns. Somatic exercises target the muscles and connective tissues surrounding the hips and pelvis, improving strength, flexibility, and coordination.

Somatic Exercise: Hip Flexor Release

The set of muscles responsible for lifting the leg. Tightness can cause discomfort, and restricted movement is known as hip flexors. Try this exercise to release tension and improve mobility.

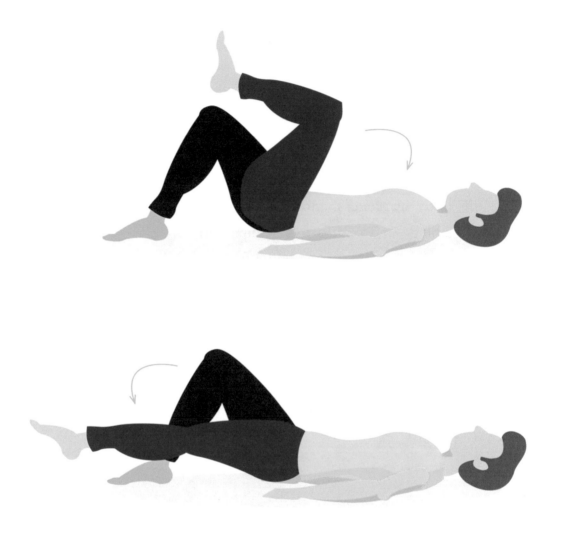

1. *Starting Position:* Lie on your back, bend your knees, keep your feet straight on the floor, and let your arms rest by your sides.

2. *Engage Abdominal Muscles:* Exhale and engage your stomach muscles to stabilize your pelvis and support your lower back.

3. *Pelvic Tilt:* Tilt your pelvis by pressing your lower back into the floor. This will lengthen your hip flexors and prepare them for release.

4. *Bring One Knee Towards Chest:* Bring one knee towards your chest while keeping the opposite foot on the floor.

5. *Extend Opposite Leg:* Extend the opposite leg straight and feel a gentle stretch along the front of the hip and thigh.

6. *Relax and Breathe:* Relax your hip flexor muscles while holding the stretch. Breathe deeply through your nose to guide yourself deeper into the stretch.

7. *Mindful Awareness:* Focus on your hip flexors and thighs. Notice any discomfort and breathe into those sensations to release the tension.

8. *Hold and Release:* Hold for 30 seconds to 1 minute, then release and repeat on your other side.

9. *Switch Legs:* Repeat the sequence on the other side, bringing the opposite knee towards your chest while extending the other leg along the floor.

10. *Complete Relaxation:* Rest in a neutral position after releasing your legs. Notice any changes in sensation.

Somatic Exercise: Pelvic Floor Activation

Pelvic floor activation exercises strengthen and engage pelvic floor muscles. They support bladder, bowel, and reproductive organs, improve their function, and reduce the risk of dysfunction.

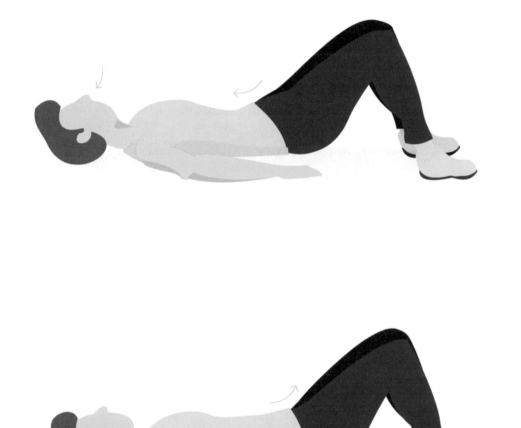

1. *Find a Comfortable Position:* Start by either sitting on a chair with your feet straight on the floor or lying down on your back with your knees bent. Keep your arms relaxed by your sides.

2. *Relax and Breathe:* Relax your body and mind. Take slow, deep breaths in and out through your nose, allowing your body to soften and relax with each exhale.

3. *Engage Your Core:* On an exhale, gently engage your stomach by drawing your belly towards your spine.

4. *Locate Your Pelvic Floor Muscles:* Close your eyes and visualize your pelvic floor muscles.

5. *Activate Your Pelvic Floor Muscles:* Squeeze and lift your pelvic floor muscles as if you were stopping urination or preventing gas passage. Lift the muscles upwards and inwards towards your navel while inhaling.

6. *Hold the Contraction:* Contract your pelvic floor muscles for 5-10 seconds, avoiding breath-holding or tensing other muscles.

7. *Release and Relax:* Relax your pelvic floor muscles and feel a sense of letting go in that area.

8. *Repeat the Activation:* Aim to repeat this at least 10-15 reps, gradually increasing the number once you become comfortable with it.

9. *Maintain Awareness:* Stay aware of your pelvic floor muscles throughout the exercise. Notice their subtle engagement and release with each contraction and relaxation.

Somatic Exercise: Hip Circles

Hip circles are a dynamic somatic exercise that helps improve mobility, flexibility, and awareness in the hips and pelvis. This exercise involves moving the hips in circular motions, which helps release tension, improve circulation, and promote relaxation in the hip joints and surrounding muscles.

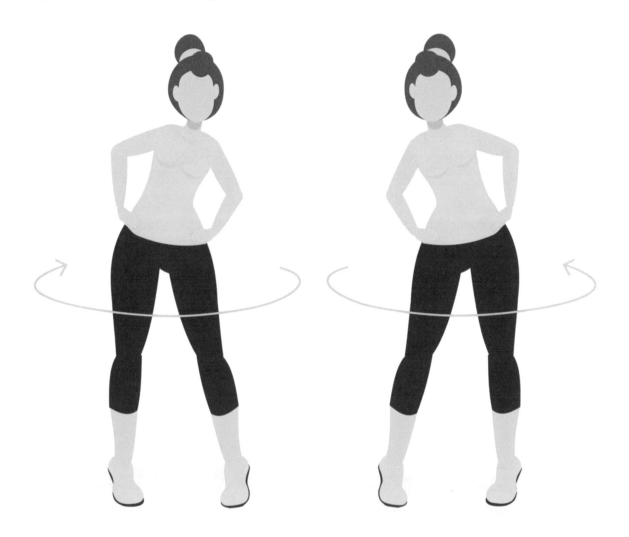

1. *Find a Comfortable Stance:* Begin by standing with your feet hip-width apart and your arms relaxed by your sides.

2. *Engage Your Core:* Gently engage your abdominal muscles by drawing your navel towards your spine.

3. *Initiate the Movement:* Shift your weight slightly to one side as you begin to circle your hips in a clockwise direction.

4. *Focus on Fluidity:* Keep your movements fluid and controlled, maintaining a steady rhythm throughout.

5. *Explore Range of Motion:* Move as far forward, to the side, back, and to the other side as feels comfortable without straining or overexerting.

6. *Coordinate with Breath:* Coordinate your hip circles with your breath, inhaling as you move your hips forward and exhaling as you move them back.

7. *Reverse the Direction:* After circling in a clockwise direction for 1-2 minutes, switch to counterclockwise circling.

8. *Maintain Alignment:* Throughout the exercise, maintain proper alignment in your spine and body posture.

9. *Focus on Sensations:* Bring your attention to the sensations in your hips and pelvis as you perform hip circles. Notice any areas of tension or restriction and adjust the intensity or range of motion accordingly.

10. *Repeat and Enjoy:* Continue for 1-2 minutes, gradually increasing the time once you become comfortable with it.

Somatic Exercise: Glute Bridge

The Glute Bridge is a fundamental somatic exercise that targets the gluteal muscles, hamstrings, and core while also promoting stability and mobility in the hips and pelvis. It helps strengthen the posterior chain muscles, improve posture, and alleviate tension in the lower back.

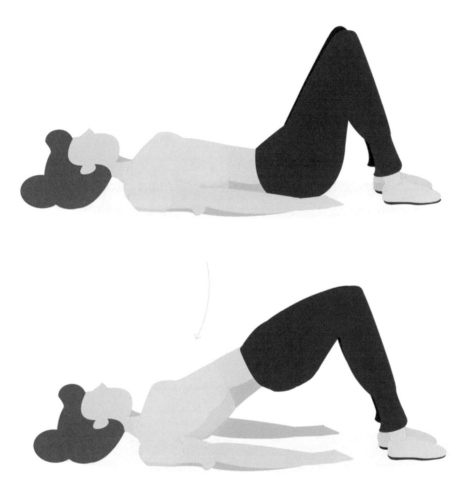

1. *Starting Position:* Start by laying on your back, bending your knees, keep your feet straight on the floor, and let your arms rest by your sides.

2. *Engage Your Core:* Gently engage your stomach by drawing your belly button towards your spine as you exhale.

3. *Press into Your Feet:* Firmly press into your feet and lift your hips towards the ceiling, engaging your glutes and hamstrings as you inhale.

4. *Lift Your Hips:* Keep lifting your hips until you form as straight line from your shoulders to your knees without overexerting yourself.

5. *Squeeze Your Glutes:* At the top of the movement, squeeze your glutes together to fully engage the muscles of your buttocks.

6. *Maintain Alignment:* Make sure to keep your hips straight on the floor throughout the exercise.

7. *Hold at the Top:* Hold for 1-2 seconds, focusing on the contraction of your glutes and the stability of your pelvis. Breathe steadily and engage your core.

8. *Lower with Control:* Slowly lower your hips back down to the starting position, vertebra by vertebra, maintaining control over the movement as you exhale.

9. *Repeat the Movement:* Aim to repeat this at least 10-15 reps, gradually increasing the number once you become comfortable with it.

Somatic Exercise: Figure 4 Stretch

The Figure 4 stretch is a simple yet effective somatic exercise that targets the muscles of the hips, glutes, and lower back. This stretch helps reduce tension, improve flexibility, and promote relaxation in the hip joints and the muscles around it.

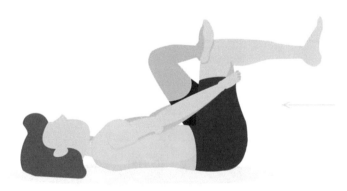

1. *Starting Position* Lie on your back, bend your knees, keep your feet flat on the floor, and let your arms rest by your sides.

2. *Engage Your Core:* Gently engage your stomach by drawing your belly button towards your spine as you exhale.as you exhale.

3. *Cross One Ankle Over Opposite Knee:* Lift one foot off the floor and cross your ankle over the opposite knee, forming a "figure 4" shape with your legs as you inhale. Flex the foot of the lifted leg to protect the knee joint.

4. *Intertwine Your Hands:* Thread your hands around the thigh of the leg with the ankle crossed over the knee.

5. *Gently Pull Knee Towards Chest:* Gently pull the knee of the crossed leg towards your chest, feeling a stretch in the hip and glute of the lifted leg as you exhale.

6. *Maintain Relaxation:* Relax your shoulders and neck, allowing your upper body to remain heavy on the mat.

7. *Feel the Stretch:* Focus on the sensation of the stretch in your hip and glute muscles. Notice any areas of tightness or restriction and breathe.

8. *Maintain Posture:* Hold the stretch for 30 seconds to 1 minute, or longer if desired, maintaining a steady and even breath pattern throughout.

9. *Switch Legs:* Release the crossed leg and return both feet to the floor. Repeat the Figure 4 stretch on the opposite side.

10. *Complete Relaxation:* Take a moment to rest in a neutral position, allowing your spine and pelvis to return to their natural alignment.

Incorporating hip and pelvic stability somatic exercises into your routine can help improve posture, balance, and overall mobility. By targeting the muscles around the hips and pelvis, these exercises promote strength, flexibility, and coordination, supporting optimal function and reducing the risk of injury.

8

CORE STRENGTHENING SOMATIC EXERCISES

In this chapter, we will learn somatic exercises designed to strengthen and stabilize the core muscles, including the abdominals and lower back. The core muscles form the foundation of the body's stability and support, providing a strong center from which all movement originates. Strengthening the core not only improves physical performance but also reduces the risk of injury and supports overall health and well-being. Somatic exercises focused on core strengthening target the deep muscles of the abdomen, pelvis, and lower back, helping to build strength, stability, and resilience from the inside out.

Somatic Exercise: Engaging the Core

Engaging the core is a fundamental somatic exercise that helps strengthen and activate the muscles of the abdomen, pelvis, and lower back. This exercise focuses on building awareness and control of the deep core muscles.

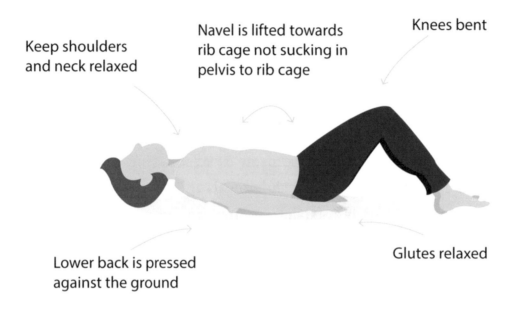

1. *Find a Comfortable Position*: Start by lying or sitting in a comfortable position with your feet flat on the floor and arms resting on your sides.

2. *Relax Your Body:* Relax your body and mind. Take slow, deep breaths in and out through your nose, allowing your body to soften and relax with each exhale.

3. *Engage Your Abdominals:* Gently engage your stomach by drawing your belly button towards your spine as you exhale. as you exhale.

4. *Activate Your Pelvic Floor:* Activate your pelvic floor muscles by drawing them upwards and inwards, as if you were trying to stop the flow of urine or prevent passing gas.

5. *Maintain the Engagement:* Hold for 5-10 seconds, maintaining a gentle but firm engagement. Keep the rest of your body relaxed and still.

6. *Breathe Normally:* Allow your breath to flow freely as you maintain the core activation.

7. *Release and Relax:* Relax your abdomen and pelvic floor muscles, and take a moment to rest and observe any sensations in your body.

8. Repeat the Activation: Aim to repeat this at least 5-10 reps, gradually increasing the number once you become comfortable with it.

Somatic Exercise: Abdominal Activation

This exercise helps improve core stability, support proper posture, and enhance overall abdominal strength and function.

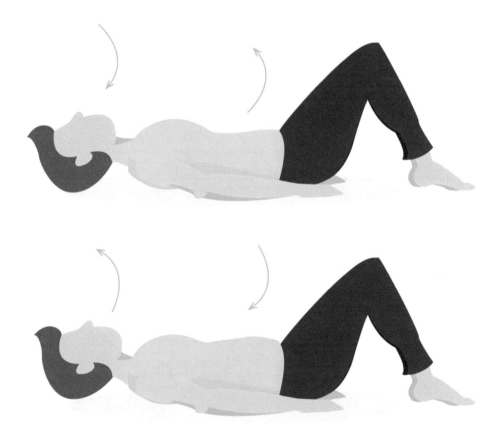

1. *Find a Comfortable Position:* Start by lying or sitting in a comfortable position with your feet flat on the floor and arms resting on your sides.

2. *Relax Your Body:* Relax your body and mind. Take slow, deep breaths in and out through your nose, allowing your body to soften and relax with each exhale.

3. *Engage Your Abdominals:* Gently engage your stomach by drawing your belly button towards your spine as you exhale as you exhale.

4. *Focus on the Lower Abdominals:* Visualize drawing these muscles inward and upward towards your spine, creating a sense of lift and engagement in the lower belly.

5. *Maintain the Engagement:* Hold for 5-10 seconds, maintaining a gentle but firm engagement.

6. *Breathe Normally:* Allow your breath to flow freely as you maintain the core activation.

7. *Release and Relax:* Relax your abdomen and pelvic floor muscles, and take a moment to rest and observe any sensations in your body.

8. *Repeat the Activation:* Aim to repeat this at least 5-10 reps, gradually increasing the number once you become comfortable with it.

Somatic Plank Variation Exercises

Plank variations are dynamic somatic exercises that target the muscles of the core, shoulders, arms, and legs. These exercises help improve core strength, stability, and endurance while also engaging multiple muscle groups throughout the body.

1. *Side Plank:* Start with your traditional plank position, then rotate onto one side, stacking your feet and shoulders. Lift your hips towards the ceiling, creating a straight line from head to heels. Hold for 30 seconds to 1 minute, then switch sides. Then, repeat for 5-10 rounds.

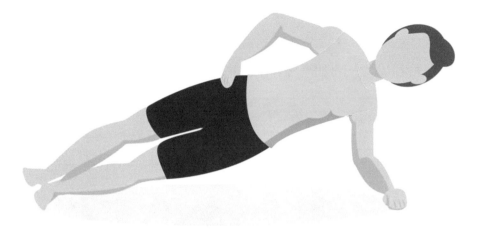

2. *Plank Shoulder Taps:* Initiate your plank position with your hands directly under your shoulders. Lift one hand off the floor, tap the opposite shoulder, and return to the starting position. Alternate sides for 10-15 repetitions.

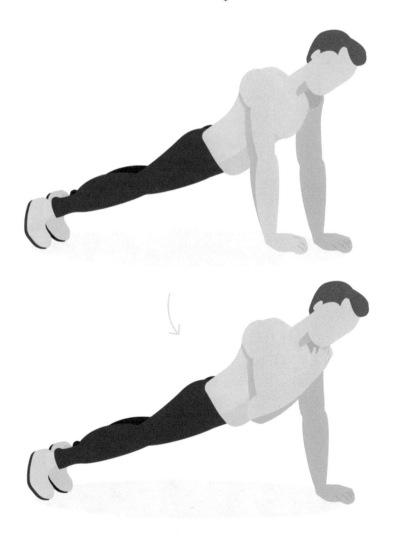

3. *Plank with Leg Lifts:* Begin in a plank position, then lift one leg off the floor, keeping it straight and engaged. Hold for a few seconds, then lower the leg back down and repeat on the opposite side. Continue for a repetition of 10-15 while alternative your legs.

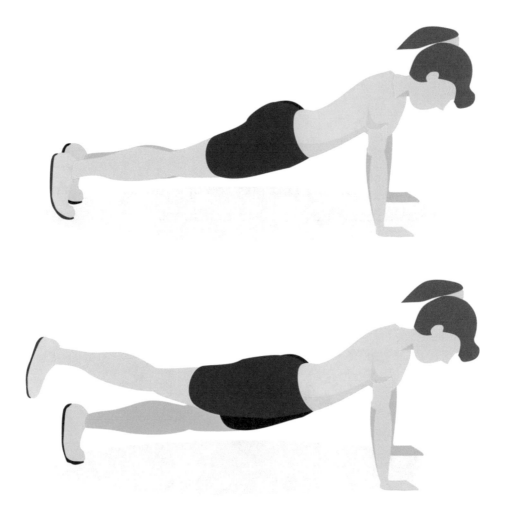

4. *Plank Knee-to-Elbow:* Start in a simple plank position, then bring one knee towards the same elbow, engaging the oblique and core muscles. Move back to the initial position you started with and repeat on the other side. Continue alternating sides for 10-15 repetitions.

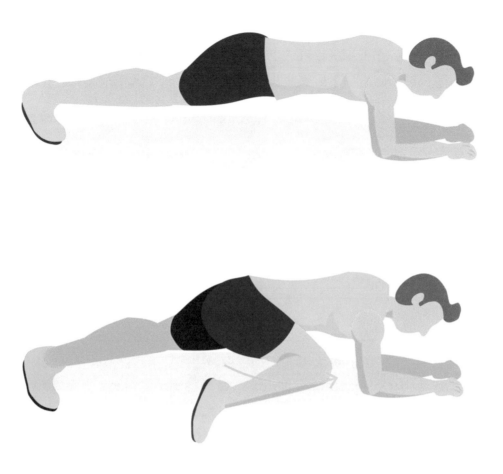

5. *Reverse Plank*: Start by sitting down on the floor with your legs extended in front of you and your hands planted on the floor behind your hips. Press in your hands and lift your hips upwards. Hold the position for 30 seconds to 1 minute. Then, repeat for 5-10 rounds.

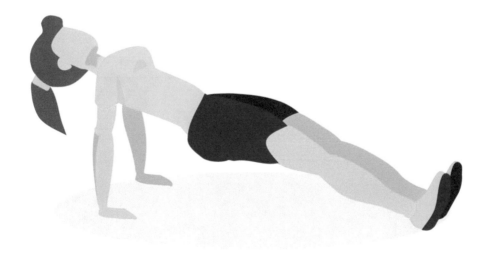

6. *Forearm Plank with Hip Dips:* Begin in a forearm plank position with your elbows directly under your shoulders. Slowly lower one hip towards the floor, then return to the starting position and lower the opposite hip. Continue alternating sides for 10-15 repetitions.

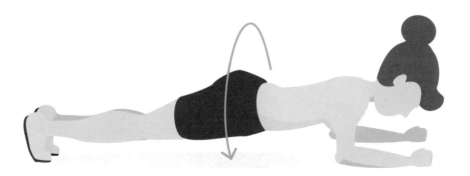

7. *Plank Jacks:* Start in a regular plank position with your feet together. Jump your feet out wide, then back together, maintaining a strong plank position throughout. Continue for 10-15 repetitions.

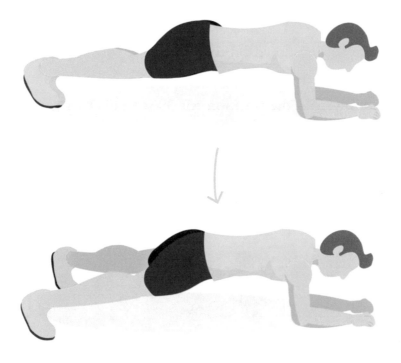

8. *High Plank with Shoulder Blade Squeeze:* Begin in a traditional plank position with your hands directly under your shoulders. Squeeze your shoulder blades together, engaging the muscles of the upper back. Hold for 10-15 seconds, then release and repeat for 5-10 rounds.

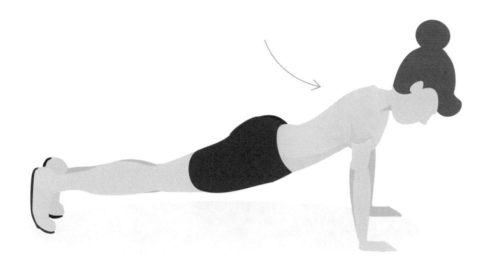

Somatic Exercise: Dead Bug

The Dead Bug exercise is a dynamic somatic exercise that targets the muscles of the core while promoting stability and mobility in the hips and shoulders. This exercise helps improve core strength, coordination, and body awareness, making it an effective addition to any fitness routine.

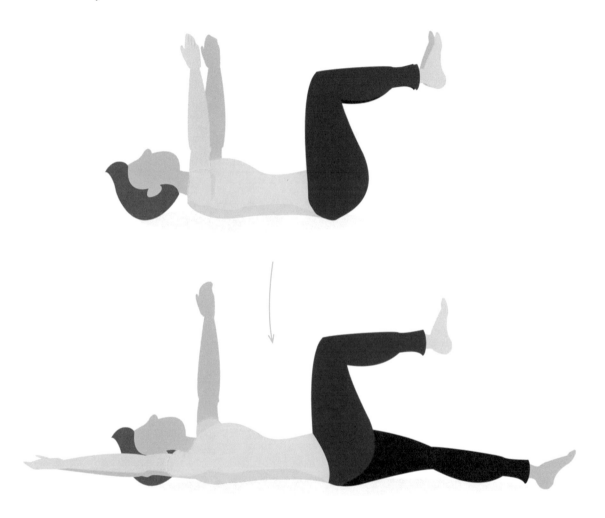

1. *Starting Position:* Comfortably lay on your back with your knees and hips bent at a 90-degree angle. With your shins parallel to the floor. Stretch out your arms upwards, directly above your shoulders, with your palms facing each other.

2. *Engage Your Core:* Gently engage your stomach by drawing your belly button towards your spine as you exhale as you exhale.

3. *Lower One Leg and Opposite Arm:* Maintain a 90-degree angle bend in your knee and hip, lowering your right arm behind you towards the floor and your left leg towards the floor in front of you.

4. *Maintain Stability:* Avoid allowing your lower back to arch or lift off the floor. Keep your abdominals engaged to support your spine and pelvis.

5. *Return to Starting Position:* Return your right arm and left leg to the starting position, bringing them back to the 90-degree position above your shoulders and hips.

6. *Alternate Sides:* Keep repeating on either side.

7. *Continue Alternating:* Continue changing sides for 10-15 repetitions on each side or as many repetitions as possible while maintaining proper form and control.

8. *Rest and Relax:* Relax your body and mind. Take slow, deep breaths in and out through your nose, allowing your body to soften and relax with each exhale.

Somatic Exercise: Russian Twist

The Russian Twist helps improve rotational strength, stability, and coordination, making it a valuable addition to any fitness routine.

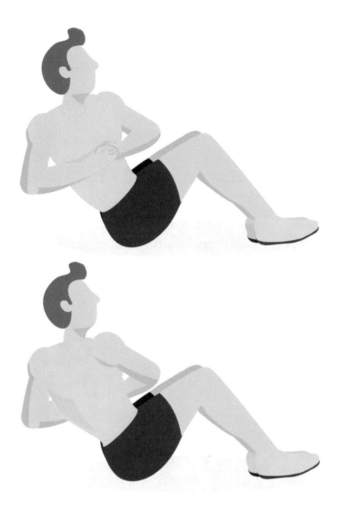

1. *Starting Position:* Sit on the floor with your knees bent and feet flat on the floor, hip-width apart, spine straight, and art extended straight in front of you, clasping together.

2. *Engage Your Core:* Gently engage your stomach by drawing your belly button towards your spine as you exhale as you exhale.

3. *Rotate Your Torso:* Rotate your torso to the right, bringing your clasped hands or weight towards the floor beside your right hip as you exhale.

4. *Pause and Hold:* Hold the rotated position for a moment, feeling the engagement of your core muscles as you maintain balance and control.

5. *Return to Center:* Slowly rotate your torso back to the center, bringing your clasped hands or weight back in front of you as you inhale.

6. *Rotate to the Opposite Side:* Repeat the rotation to the left side, bringing your clasped hands or weight towards the floor beside your left hip.

7. *Pause and Hold:* Hold the rotated position for a moment, maintaining balance and control while feeling the engagement of your core muscles.

8. *Repeat the Movement:* Aim for 10-15 repetitions on each side or as many repetitions as possible while maintaining proper form and control.

9. *Complete the Set:* Relax your body and mind. Take slow, deep breaths in and out through your nose, allowing your body to soften and relax with each exhale.

Core strengthening somatic exercises are essential to any fitness routine, supporting overall strength, stability, and mobility. Incorporating these exercises into your regular practice can improve posture, reduce the risk of injury, and enhance performance in everyday activities and exercise. Practice these core strengthening exercises mindfully and consistently to experience the benefits of a strong and resilient core for optimal health and well-being.

Chapter 9

SOMATIC EXERCISES FOR BALANCE AND PROPRIOCEPTION

This chapter will explore a series of somatic exercises designed to improve balance and proprioception, enhancing your body's ability to sense its position and movement in space.

Balance refers to the ability to maintain equilibrium and stability while standing, walking, or performing other activities, while proprioception is the sense that enables us to perceive the position, orientation, and movement of our body parts relative to one another and the environment.

Somatic Exercise: Single Leg Stance

The Single Leg Stance is a foundational somatic exercise that enhances balance, stability, and proprioception while also strengthening the muscles of the lower body and core. It is particularly beneficial for improving functional movement patterns and reducing the risk of falls and injuries.

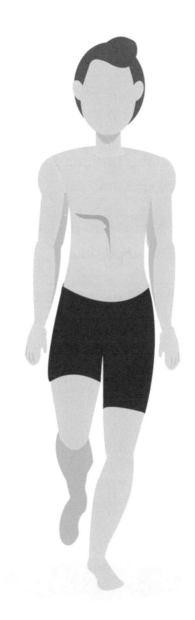

1. *Starting Position:* Begin by standing tall with your feet hip-width apart and your arms relaxed by your sides.

2. *Engage Your Core:* Gently engage your stomach by drawing your belly button towards your spine as you exhale as you exhale.

3. *Shift Your Weight:* Move the weight of your body onto one foot, lifting the opposite foot slightly off the floor. Keep a slight bend in the knee of your left support.

4. *Maintain Balance:* Focus on maintaining balance and stability on the single supporting leg.

5. *Stabilize Your Hips:* Engage the muscles of your hip, particularly the glutes and hip abductors, to stabilize your pelvis and prevent it from tilting or dropping to one side.

6. *Hold the Position:* Hold yourself in this position for 15-30 seconds, or as long as you can maintain proper form and control.

7. *Switch Sides:* Repeat the single-leg stance on the other side, focusing on maintaining balance and stability with the new supporting leg.

8. *Complete the Set:* Aim for 3-5 repetitions on each side, or as many repetitions as possible, while maintaining proper form and control.

Somatic Exercise: Fashion Walk

The Heel-to-Toe Walk is a somatic exercise designed to improve balance, coordination, and proprioception by challenging your body's ability to maintain stability while walking in a straight line. This exercise helps you strengthen the muscles of the lower body and core, promotes proper posture, and enhances overall body awareness.

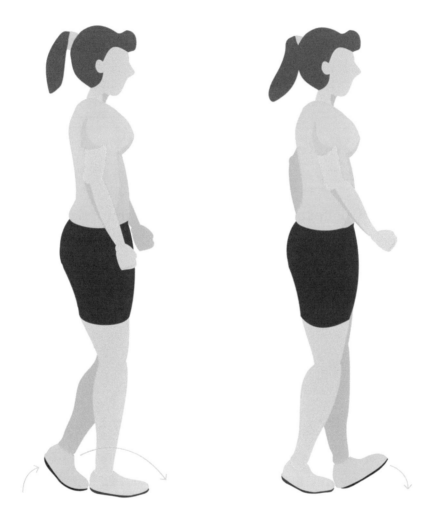

1. *Find a Clear Path:* Find a clear, flat surface to walk on, such as a hallway or open space. Make sure there are no obstacles or hazards in your path.

2. *Stand Tall:* Stand tall with your feet together and your arms relaxed by your sides.

3. *Start Walking:* Take a step forward with your right foot, placing your right heel directly in front of the toes of your left foot. Focus on placing your right heel precisely in line with the toes of your left foot, creating a straight line with your feet.

4. *Transfer Weight:* Shift your weight onto your right foot as you roll forward onto the ball of your foot. Maintain balance and stability as you transfer your weight from your left foot to your right foot.

5. *Continue Walking:* Take a step forward with your left foot, placing your left heel directly in front of the toes of your right foot.

6. *Shift Weight:* Maintain balance and stability as you transfer your weight from your right foot to your left foot.

7. *Repeat the Process:* Continue walking in a straight line, alternating steps between your right and left foot.

8. *Maintain Posture:* Keep your gaze fixed ahead of you and your chest lifted throughout the exercise.

9. *Complete the Walk:* Continue for 10-20 steps, or as far as your space allows. Maintain balance, stability, and proper alignment with each step.

Somatic Exercises with Balance Pad

Balance pads are versatile tools that can enhance balance, stability, and proprioception through somatic exercises. Incorporating balance pad exercises into your routine can improve functional movement patterns, reduce the risk of falls, and enhance overall body awareness and control.

1. *Standing Balance on Balance Pad:* Stand on the balance pad with your feet hip-width apart, engage your core muscles, and maintain a tall, upright posture. Hold the standing position for 30 seconds to 1 minute, or as long as you can maintain stability and control.

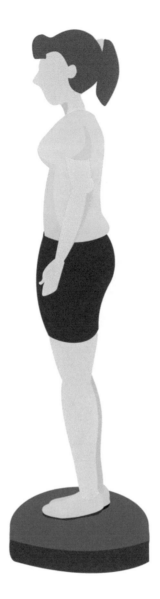

2. *Single-Leg Balance on Balance Pad:* Stand on the balance pad with one foot centered on the pad and the other foot lifted slightly off the ground. Engage your core muscles and maintain balance. Hold for 15-30 seconds, then switch sides and repeat for 10-15 repetitions.

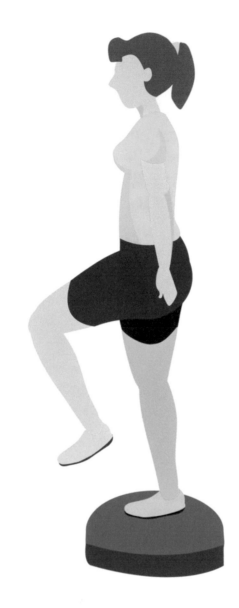

3. *Squats on Balance Pad:* Stand on the balance pad and your arms extended in front of you. Lower into a squat position by bending your knees and hips, keeping your weight centered over the middle of the pad. Press through your heels to return to the starting position, engaging your glutes and quadriceps. Perform 10-15 repetitions of squats on the balance pad, maintaining stability.

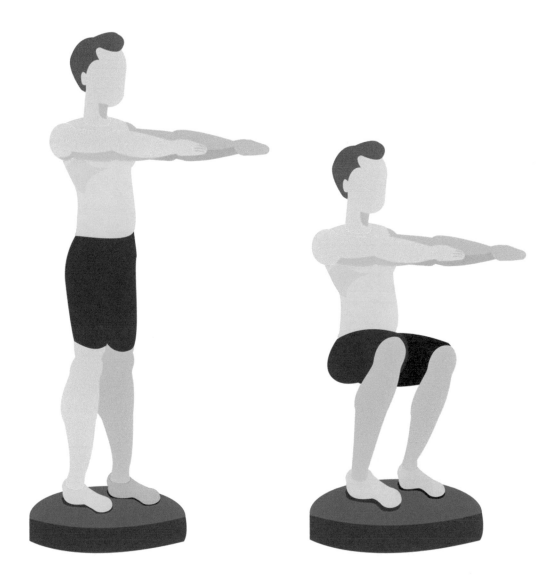

4. *Lunges on Balance Pad:* Stand on the balance pad with your feet hip-width apart and your hands on your hips. Step one foot back into a lunge position, placing the ball of your back foot on the pad. Lower your back knee towards the ground, keeping your front knee aligned with your toes and torso upright. Press through your front heel to return to the starting position, engaging your quadriceps and glutes. Perform 10-15 repetitions of lunges on each leg, focusing on maintaining balance and stability on the pad.

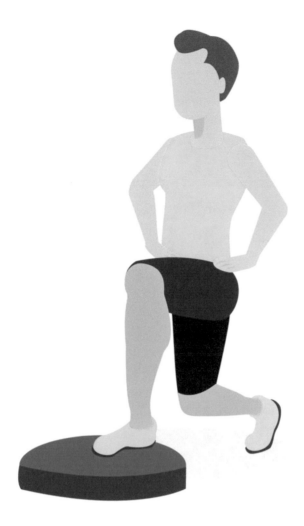

5. *Plank on Balance Pad:* Begin in a plank position with your hands directly under your shoulders and your toes on the balance pad. Engage your core muscles and keep your body in a straight line from head to heels, avoiding any sagging or arching in the lower back. Hold the plank position for 30 seconds to 1 minute, focusing on maintaining stability and control on the unstable surface. To increase the challenge, try lifting one foot off the pad or tapping your knees on the pad while maintaining the plank position.

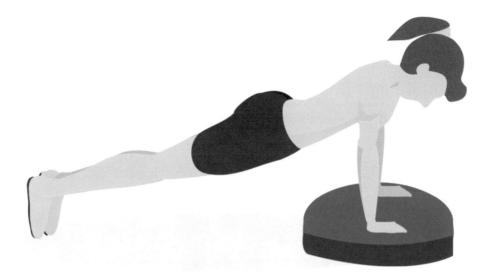

6. *Seated Balance Exercises on Balance Pad:* Sit on the balance pad with your legs crossed or extended in front of you. Engage your core muscles and sit tall, balancing on the pad without using your hands for support. Hold the seated balance position for 30 seconds to 1 minute, focusing on maintaining stability and control. To increase the challenge, try closing your eyes or lifting one foot off the pad while maintaining balance in the seated position.

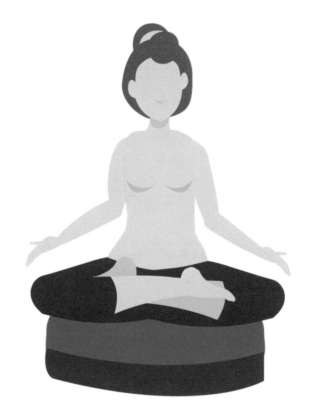

Somatic Exercise: Standing Leg Raises

Standing leg raises are dynamic somatic exercises that target the muscles of the lower body, particularly the hips, thighs, and glutes. This exercise improves balance, stability, and proprioception while strengthening the hip abduction and flexion muscles.

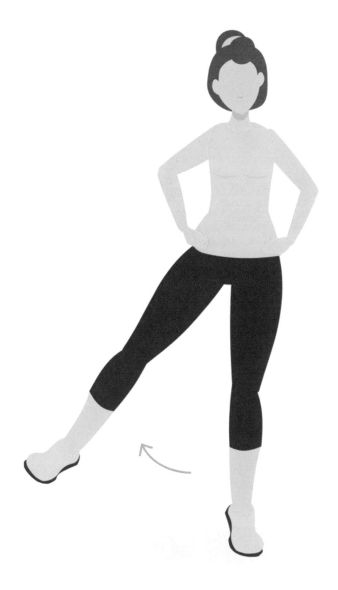

1. *Starting Position:* Begin by standing tall with your feet hip-width apart and your arms relaxed by your sides.

2. *Engage Your Core:* Gently engage your stomach by drawing your belly button towards your spine as you exhale as you exhale.

3. *Shift Your Weight:* Shift your weight onto one leg while keeping a slight bend in the knee of your supporting leg.

4. *Lift the Opposite Leg:* Lift the opposite leg out to the side, keeping it straight and engaged as you inhale. Lift the leg as high as possible while maintaining stability and control.

5. *Pause and Hold:* Hold the lifted position for a moment, focusing on engaging the muscles of the outer thigh and hip to lift the leg.

6. *Lower the Leg:* Lower the lifted leg back down to the starting position with control as you exhale.

7. *Switch Sides:* Repeat the exercise on the opposite leg, shifting your weight onto the other leg and lifting the opposite leg out to the side.

8. *Complete the Set:* Aim for 10-15 repetitions on each side or as many repetitions as you can while maintaining proper form and control.

Somatic Exercise: Tree Pose

Tree Pose is a classic yoga posture that can be adapted into a somatic exercise to improve balance, stability, and body awareness. This pose helps in strengthening the muscles of the legs and core while also promoting relaxation and focus.

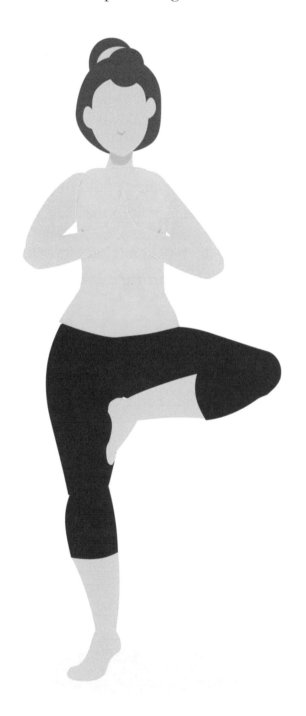

1. *Starting Position:* Begin by standing tall with your feet hip-width apart and your arms relaxed by your sides.

2. *Shift Your Weight:* Shift your weight onto your left foot and ground down through the sole of your foot.

3. *Lift Your Right Foot:* Fold your right knee and bring the sole of your right foot on the inside of your left thigh to rest.

4. *Find Your Balance:* Press your right foot in your left thigh and your left thigh into your right foot to create a stable foundation and keep your core engaged.

5. *Bring Your Hands to Heart Center:* Press your palms together and bring them in front of your chest in a prayer position.

6. *Lengthen Your Spine:* Lengthen your spine by lifting the crown of your head towards the ceiling and drawing your shoulders down and away from your ears.

7. *Hold the Pose:* Hold this pose between 30 seconds and 1 minute, or as long as you can maintain balance and stability.

8. *Release and Repeat:* Release the pose by gently lowering your right foot back down to the floor and returning to a standing position with both feet hip-width apart.

9. *Switch Sides:* Repeat the same sequence on the opposite side, shifting your weight onto your right foot and bringing your left foot to rest on the inside of your right thigh.

By incorporating these exercises into your routine regularly, you can enhance your sense of balance, reduce the risk of falls and injuries, and improve functional movement patterns in everyday life.

Chapter 10

INTEGRATING SOMATIC INTO DAILY LIFE

This chapter will discuss the practical strategies for integrating somatic exercises and principles into your daily routine to promote health, well-being, and vitality. Somatic is not your standard set of exercises; it's a way of living with a mindful connection with your body and inner self. Practicing these exercises daily can enhance your physical, mental, and emotional resilience and help you experience greater ease and joy in all you do.

Postural Awareness

Postural awareness is vital in incorporating somatic exercises into your daily lives. It involves paying attention to your body's natural state and how you hold it in various positions throughout the day. It can include awareness of alignment, muscle tension, and movement patterns. By practicing developing postural awareness, we can identify and correct habits that may contribute to postural problems and body aches.

Tips for Postural Awareness

1. **Be mindful of your body** and take note of your posture throughout the day. If you notice any misalignment or areas of tension, make sure to fix your posture accordingly.

2. Incorporate **gentle stretches and exercises throughout the day**, such as shoulder rolls, chest openers, and spine twists, to help release tension and improve your posture.

3. Use **verbal cues** to bring attention to your posture and make adjustments when required. Cues such as "lengthen the spine" and "soften the shoulders" will help you become mindful of that specific body part.

4. Try to **incorporate mindfulness techniques**, such as body scanning meditation, to help deepen your awareness of physical sensations and alignment.

Ergonomics in Daily Activities

The science of designing and arranging things in the environment to fit the capabilities and limitations of the human body is known as ergonomics. In Somatic, ergonomics means more than just the design of physical objects; it encompasses how we move and interact with our environment in everyday activities. Suppose we apply the principle of bodily exercises to ergonomics. In that case, we can optimize our movements and posture, which will improve the level of comfort, efficiency, and well-being of our daily lives. Here is a list of somatic exercises that can help you enhance ergonomics in your various daily activities:

1. *Sitting at a Desk:* Many people spend countless hours sitting at their desks, whether at work, home, or school, which can lead to discomfort and strain in the neck, shoulders, and back. Somatic exercises can reduce the amount of tension and promote better posture while sitting. You can use somatic techniques to improve posture while sitting, such as pelvic tilts and spinal twists, to maintain alignment and reduce strain on the lower back.

2. *Standing and Walking:* Standing and walking are fundamental activities in our daily lives that can benefit from ergonomic adjustments to promote comfort and ease of movement. Incorporating somatic exercises that can improve alignment and balance while standing, such as grounding through the feet and lengthening through the spine, will help release tension and stress in your body. You can use

somatic techniques to enhance the quality of movement while walking, such as mindful walking exercises that focus on the sensation of each step.

3. *Lifting and Carrying:* Lifting and carrying objects can strain the body if not done using proper technique and alignment. You can start by practicing somatic exercises that help activate the core and stabilize the spine before lifting heavy objects, such as pelvic floor engagement and abdominal bracing, using somatic techniques to maintain alignment and distribute weight evenly while carrying objects, such as lengthening through the spine and engaging the shoulders and arms with awareness.

4. *Using Electronic Devices:* If not done mindfully, electronic devices can contribute to poor posture and muscular tension. By using somatic exercises, you can help reduce these effects and promote the ergonomic use of electronic devices. Daily practice of somatic exercises can help to release tension in the neck, shoulders, and wrists caused by prolonged use of electronic devices, such as gentle stretches and self-massage techniques.

Tips for Ergonomics in Daily Activities

1. Try setting up your workspace ergonomically, with a chair with good postural support, a desk at an appropriate height, and computer equipment positioned to minimize strain on the neck and shoulders.

2. Using ergonomic tools and accessories, such as an ergonomic keyboard and mouse, can promote comfortable and efficient work habits.

3. Make minor environmental adjustments to support proper posture during activities like driving, cooking, and watching TV, using cushions or supports as needed.

4. Make sure to take regular breaks to stretch and move throughout the day and avoid prolonged periods of sitting or standing in one position.

Including somatic exercises in daily activities can help you cultivate a greater awareness of movement habits and make ergonomic adjustments to promote comfort, efficiency, and well-being. By using mindful attention and practice techniques, we can optimize our movements and posture to support the health and vitality of our bodies in all aspects of daily life.

Mindful Sitting and Standing

Practicing mindful sitting and standing involves bringing awareness to the sensations and alignment of the body while performing these essential activities. Incorporating mindfulness during sitting and standing can help to reduce tension, improve posture, and cultivate a sense of ease and presence in our bodies.

Tips for Mindful Sitting and Standing

1. Take a moment to check your body before sitting or standing, and notice any areas of tension or discomfort.

2. Be mindful every time you sit and stand while also paying attention to the alignment of your spine, pelvis, and shoulders. You can also keep your core engaged to improve your posture and balance.

3. Switch to mindful breathing techniques and take deep and slow breaths to improve your awareness and comfort.

4. Use slow and deliberate movement to help maintain body awareness by transitioning between sitting and standing.

Including somatic practices in your everyday routine can be a constructive way to cultivate greater awareness, presence, and vitality. By embracing mindfulness, movement, and self-care as essential parts of your life, you can develop a deep sense of connection with yourself and the world around you. As you continue to explore and embody Somatic, may you find new opportunities for growth, healing, and happiness.

Chapter

11

STRESS MANAGEMENT THROUGH SOMATIC AND MINDFULNESS PRACTICES

In this chapter, we will discuss how Somatic techniques and mindfulness practices can help manage stress, promote relaxation, and develop greater resilience to challenges you face in life. With regular use of somatic awareness and mindfulness techniques in our daily routine, we can learn to respond to stress more easily and clearly, leading to better overall health and quality of life.

Understanding Stress

In life, we all face situations that can trigger stress. This can be due to the challenges we encounter or the perceived threats around us. Stress is a natural response that activates the body's "fight or flight" response, which can be beneficial in the short term. However, chronic stress can have a negative impact on our overall health, leading to various mental, emotional, and physical health problems, such as anxiety, depression, and cardiovascular disease. Therefore, it is crucial to manage stress effectively to maintain a healthy and fulfilling life.

Somatic Techniques for Stress Management

Somatic techniques provide a comprehensive solution for managing stress, emphasizing the vital link between the mind and body and encouraging relaxation and self-control. By engaging in somatic exercises, we can eliminate stress-causing tension, diminish the physiological stress response, and foster an increased sense of tranquility and wellness.

1. *Body Scan Meditation:* Start by practicing a body scan meditation to enhance awareness of the body and tension in the body. Start by bringing attention to each area of the body, from head to toe, noticing any areas of tightness or discomfort. With each breath, allow these sensations to soften and release, promoting relaxation and stress relief.

2. *Progressive Muscle Relaxation:* This technique involves equal tensing and relaxing different sets of muscles in the body to promote relaxation and reduce stress. Begin by tensing a specific muscle group for a few seconds, such as the shoulders or fists, then release and relax the muscles completely. Move through each muscle group, noticing the sensation of relaxation spreading throughout the body.

3. *Diaphragmatic Breathing:* Also known as belly breathing, it involves deep, slow breathing while keeping the diaphragm engaged and promotes relaxation of the nervous system. Practice this technique by placing one hand on your belly and the other on your chest. Start by deeply breathing in through your nose, allowing your belly to rise as you fill your lungs with air, then slowly breathe out through your mouth, feeling your belly relax. Repeat this process for several breaths, focusing on the sensation of relaxation with each exhale.

4. *Mindful Movement Practices:* Use mindful movement practices, such as yoga, tai chi, or qigong, to promote relaxation, flexibility, and body awareness. These practices combine gentle movement, breathwork, and mindfulness to reduce stress and promote a sense of calm and well-being. Focus on the sensations of movement in your body, cultivating present-moment awareness and letting go of tension and anxiety with each mindful breath and movement.

5. *Grounding Techniques:* Use grounding techniques to connect with the present moment and anchor yourself in times of stress. Focus on sensory experiences, such as feeling the texture of an object in your hand, listening to the sounds around you, or noticing the sensation of your feet on the ground. Grounding techniques help

shift your focus away from stressors and promote a sense of stability and security in the present moment.

Mindfulness Practices for Stress Relief

Practicing mindfulness is a powerful technique for stress relief, promoting relaxation, mental clarity, and emotional resilience. By cultivating present-moment awareness and nonjudgmental acceptance of our thoughts, feelings, and sensations, mindfulness helps us respond to stress with greater ease and stability. Here are some mindfulness practices tailored explicitly for stress relief:

1. *Mindful Breathing:* Take a few moments to focus on your breath, paying attention to the sensations of inhalation and exhalation. Take note of the rise and fall of your chest or the expansion and contraction of your abdomen with each breath. Allow your breath to become slower and more profound, promoting relaxation and calming the nervous system.

2. *Body Scan Meditation:* Practice a body scan meditation to systematically bring awareness to different parts of your body, from head to toe. Notice any areas of tension or discomfort, and with each breath, allow these sensations to soften and release. Move through each part of the body with curiosity and compassion, promoting relaxation and stress relief.

3. *Mindful Walking:* Take a mindful walk, paying attention to the sensations of movement in your body and the environment around you. Notice the feeling of your feet touching the ground, the rhythm of your steps, and the sights and sounds of your surroundings. With each step, bring your attention back to the present moment, letting go of worries and distractions.

4. *Guided Imagery:* Engage in guided imagery exercises to evoke relaxation and calm. Close your eyes and imagine yourself in a peaceful and serene environment, such as a beach, forest, or mountaintop. Use all your senses to immerse yourself in the scene, noticing the sights, sounds, smells, and sensations around you. Allow yourself to experience a sense of tranquility and well-being in this imagined space.

5. *Loving-Kindness Meditation:* Practice loving-kindness meditation to cultivate compassion and goodwill towards yourself and others. Start by repeating positive affirmations towards yourself, silently repeating phrases such as "May I be happy, may I be healthy, may I be safe, may I be at ease." Then, extend these wishes to loved ones, acquaintances, and even those with whom you may have difficulty. Cultivating a sense of connection and kindness can counteract feelings of stress and promote emotional well-being.

6. *Mindful Eating:* Practice mindful eating by bringing full attention to the experience of eating without distractions. Notice the colors, textures, and flavors of your food and the sensations of chewing and swallowing. Eat slowly and savor each bite, tuning into your body's hunger and fullness cues. Mindful eating can help reduce stress-related eating habits and promote a greater sense of satisfaction and enjoyment in meals.

7. *Mindfulness in Daily Activities:* Bring mindfulness to everyday activities such as washing dishes, brushing your teeth, or showering. Take note of every sensation, movement, and action involved in each activity without judgment or attachment. By infusing mindfulness into daily routines, you can turn mundane tasks into opportunities for relaxation and presence.

Imagine feeling a greater sense of calm, clarity, and resilience in the face of everyday stress. By incorporating mindfulness practices into your daily life, this can become a reality. Whether through focused breathing, body awareness, guided imagery, or acts of kindness, mindfulness provides a pathway to inner peace and well-being. By embracing mindfulness, you can navigate stress with greater ease and find moments of joy and contentment amidst life's challenges. So why not start nurturing a mindful approach to life today?

12

LONG-TERM BENEFITS OF SOMATIC EXERCISES

In this chapter, we will further discuss the captivating world of Somatic and discover the remarkable and enduring advantages of incorporating somatic exercises into your daily routine. Somatic is a form of exercise that surpasses traditional physical workouts by focusing on the connection between the mind and the body, encouraging all-encompassing well-being, and sustaining long-term health and energy. By practicing somatic exercises on a regular basis, you can encounter a diverse array of benefits that stretch way beyond just the physical level.

Preventing Injury and Improving Mobility with Somatic Exercises

Somatic exercises provide a comprehensive approach to preventing injuries and improving mobility. They target the root causes of dysfunction and highlight optimal movement patterns. Practicing Somatic helps develop a better understanding of the body, reduces tension, and restores balance. By incorporating Somatic into their routine, you can minimize the risk of injury, become more flexible, and move with greater ease. Let's explore how somatic exercises contribute to preventing injuries and improving mobility.

1. *Addressing Muscle Imbalances:* Somatic exercises are a form of physical therapy that aims to diagnose and correct muscle imbalances frequently implicated in injury and restricted mobility. Unilateral or repetitive movements, poor posture, and other factors can make certain muscles tight and overused while others become weak and

underused. Somatic utilizes a series of gentle movements and stretching techniques to release tension in tight muscles and activate underused muscles, thereby restoring balance to the body and promoting more efficient movement patterns. By doing so, Somatic can reduce the risk of overuse injuries, alleviate pain and discomfort, and improve overall physical performance.

2. *Promoting Proper Alignment:* Maintaining proper alignment is crucial for the optimal functioning of our body. Misalignment can cause compensatory movements and put extra stress on our body, leading to injury. Somatic exercises are a great way to align our spine, pelvis, and joints for better biomechanics and reduced risk of injury. We can distribute forces evenly across our body with Somatic, minimizing wear and tear on our joints and soft tissues. By practicing Somatic, we can achieve better alignment and improve our overall physical health.

3. *Enhancing Flexibility and Range of Motion:* It is important to maintain good flexibility and mobility to reduce the risk of injuries and improve overall physical well-being. These exercises are used to improve the flexibility and mobility of your body by releasing tension in tight muscles and improving joint mobility. By performing these exercises, one can increase their flexibility and range of motion, reducing stiffness and allowing for more fluid movements, ultimately lowering the risk of strains, sprains, and other soft tissue injuries.

4. *Improving Body Awareness and Proprioception:* Somatic exercises are designed to help you better understand your body and its movements. They focus on cultivating greater body awareness and proprioception, which is the sense of how your body is positioned in space. By tuning into your body's various sensations and movements, you can more easily detect and correct any imbalances or dysfunctional patterns before they lead to injury. This increased awareness also improves coordination and balance, which can reduce the risk of falls and other accidents. By incorporating somatic exercises into your routine, you can gain a greater appreciation for your body and its capabilities.

5. *Releasing Chronic Tension and Stress:* When we experience chronic tension and stress, it tends to accumulate in the body, leading to muscle tightness, restricted mobility,

and increased vulnerability to injuries. Another way to reduce this tension is through regular practice of somatic exercises. Somatic involves mindful movements that aim to activate the body's relaxation response, which, in turn, helps calm the nervous system. By releasing the stored tension and promoting relaxation, Somatic reduces both physical and emotional stressors that can lead to injuries and impaired mobility. The result is a more balanced and harmonious mind-body state, which enhances the overall quality of life.

6. *Supporting Functional Movement Patterns:* Somatic exercises are designed to replicate the movements we perform during our daily routine, such as twisting, bending, and reaching. These exercises aim to improve our body's ability to execute these movements safely and effectively by emphasizing proper alignment and mindful practice. Incorporating somatic exercises into your routine can significantly reduce your risk of injury during daily activities and recreational pursuits while enhancing your overall physical capabilities.

By incorporating Somatic exercises into your daily routine, you can take a proactive approach to injury prevention and mobility improvement. Somatic exercises can address muscle imbalances, promote proper alignment, enhance flexibility and range of motion, and cultivate greater body awareness and stress relief. By mindfully and consistently practicing Somatic, you can significantly reduce the risk of injury, move with greater ease and efficiency, and enjoy a higher quality of life with improved mobility and physical resilience.

Enhancing Body Awareness and Mindfulness

Somatic practice emphasizes enhancing bodily awareness and mindfulness to promote overall physical, mental, and emotional well-being. This involves developing a heightened sense of connection with our bodies and tuning into the present moment with awareness and acceptance. By doing so, we can experience a range of benefits, including greater clarity of thought, increased resilience, and a heightened sense of vitality. In essence, Somatic exercises are designed to help us better understand our bodies and minds, fostering a deeper sense of self-awareness and promoting greater overall health and well-being.

1. *Sensory Awareness:* Somatic exercises encourage us to tune into the sensations of our bodies, including tension, relaxation, warmth, and movement. By bringing attention to these sensory experiences without judgment or attachment, we can deepen our awareness of the present moment and the subtle nuances of our physical sensations.

2. *Movement Mindfulness:* Mindful movement is a cornerstone of Somatic practice, emphasizing awareness of movement patterns, alignment, and breath. By moving slowly and deliberately, we can explore the range of motion in our joints, engage muscles mindfully, and notice how our bodies respond to different movements. Through mindful movement, we can cultivate greater coordination, balance, and grace in our movements.

3. *Breath Awareness:* The breath is a powerful anchor for mindfulness, serving as a bridge between the body and mind. Somatic exercises often incorporate breath awareness techniques to promote relaxation, regulate the nervous system, and deepen our connection with the present moment. By focusing on the rhythm of our breath, we can quiet the mind, reduce stress, and enhance bodily awareness.

4. *Body Scan Meditation:* Body scan meditation is a mindfulness practice that involves systematically bringing awareness to different parts of the body, from head to toe. By scanning the body with gentle attention and curiosity, we can notice areas of tension, discomfort, or ease and cultivate a sense of acceptance and compassion toward our bodies. Body scan meditation promotes relaxation, reduces stress, and enhances bodily awareness.

5. *Grounding Techniques:* Grounding techniques help anchor us in the present moment and connect with the sensations of our bodies. Somatic exercises often incorporate grounding techniques, such as feeling the support of the earth beneath our feet, noticing the contact points between our body and the ground, or visualizing roots extending from our body into the world. By grounding ourselves in this way, we can reduce anxiety, promote relaxation, and enhance our sense of stability and security.

Somatic practice is a technique that can help you improve your bodily awareness and mindfulness. This approach can lead to increased well-being and vitality by helping you become more aware of your body movements and breathing. It can also help you reduce stress levels and relax. Practicing Somatic regularly and living mindfully can help you tap into the wisdom of your body and find more joy, ease, and fulfillment in your day-to-day life.

30-DAY SOMATIC EXERCISE PLAN FOR BEGINNERS

Week 1: Introduction to Somatic

Day 1:

1. Begin with a gentle introduction to basic somatic principles.

2. Start with deep breathing exercises to center yourself and cultivate awareness of your breath.

3. Follow with simple bodily movements such as shoulder rolls, neck stretches, and gentle spinal twists.

4. Spend 15 minutes exploring these movements mindfully, paying attention to how your body responds.

Day 2-3:

1. Continue with deep breathing exercises, gradually extending the duration to 5-10 minutes.

2. Explore additional somatic movements focusing on different body areas, such as wrist circles, ankle rolls, and hip rotations.

3. Take time to notice any sensations or tensions in your body as you move and breathe.

Day 4-5:

1. Introduce the practice of body scan meditation, starting with a 5-minute session.

2. Follow with a series of progressive muscle relaxation exercises, systematically releasing tension from head to toe.

3. Incorporate gentle somatic movements to unwind further and release tension, allowing your body to move with greater ease and freedom.

Week 2: Body Scan and Relaxation

Day 6-8:

1. Dedicate 10-15 minutes each day to body scan meditation, gradually increasing the duration to 10-15 minutes.

2. Follow with progressive muscle relaxation techniques, focusing on areas of tension identified during the body scan.

3. Engage in gentle somatic movements to integrate the relaxation response into your body and promote a sense of overall well-being.

Day 9-10:

1. Experiment with different breathing techniques such as diaphragmatic breathing, square breathing, or alternate nostril breathing.

2. Explore how different breathing patterns affect your body and mind, and choose the technique that resonates most with you.

3. Continue to incorporate somatic movements to enhance relaxation and body awareness.

Day 11-12:

1. Deepen your somatic practice by exploring variations of familiar movements, such as adding gentle twists or extensions to traditional stretches.

2. Focus on moving with fluidity and grace, allowing your breath to guide your movements and deepen your awareness.

3. Take time to rest and integrate the benefits of your practice, noticing any shifts in your body and mind.

Week 3: Mobility and Flexibility

Day 13-15:

1. Begin to explore mobility and flexibility exercises, starting with simple movements to loosen up the joints and increase the range of motion.

2. Focus on movements that target areas of stiffness or tightness in your body, such as hip openers, shoulder stretches, and spinal twists.

3. Use your breath to support and enhance your movements, breathing deeply into areas of tension to encourage release and relaxation.

Day 16-18:

1. Further practice somatic movements that promote mobility and flexibility, incorporating dynamic stretching techniques such as gentle bouncing or pulsing movements.

2. Pay attention to your body's feedback as you move, adjusting the intensity and range of motion to suit your comfort level.

3. Take breaks as needed to rest and integrate the benefits of your practice, allowing your body to adapt and respond to the movements.

Day 19-20:

1. Explore mindful walking or moving meditation to integrate somatic principles into everyday activities.

2. Focus on moving with awareness and intention, noticing the sensations of each step and how your body interacts with the environment.

3. Reflect on how somatic awareness can be applied to daily movements and activities, bringing mindfulness and presence to each moment.

Week 4: Mindful Integration

Day 21-23:

1. Dedicate time each day to mindful integration practices, such as mindful eating, mindful listening, or mindful communication.

2. Apply somatic principles of awareness and presence to these activities, noticing how they deepen your connection with yourself and others.

3. Use gentle somatic movements as a way to ground and center yourself throughout the day, bringing awareness to your body and breathing in each moment.

Day 24-26:

1. Reflect on the past three weeks, noticing any changes or shifts in your body, mind, and spirit.

2. Set intentions for continued growth and exploration in your somatic practice, identifying areas where you would like to focus your attention and energy.

3. Take time to celebrate your progress and acknowledge your dedication and commitment to your well-being.

Day 27-30:

1. Integrate all aspects of your somatic practice into a daily routine that supports your physical, mental, and emotional well-being.

2. Continue to explore new movements, techniques, and practices that resonate with you, remaining open to the ever-evolving nature of your somatic journey.

3. Trust in the wisdom of your body and the transformative power of somatic to guide you toward more excellent health, vitality, and presence in your life.

As you follow this 30-day somatic plan, always remember to listen to your body and be mindful of its needs and limitations. This is a journey of self-discovery and exploration, and there is no single right or wrong way to practice. Embrace curiosity, keep an open mind, and fully allow yourself to experience each moment. By doing so, you'll be able to transform and benefit from this journey fully.

CONCLUSION

Dear reader,

I want to express my heartfelt gratitude to you for joining me on this journey of self-discovery. Together, we have explored the fascinating relationship between our minds and bodies and have discovered the powerful benefits of somatic exercises for our overall well-being.

Your dedication to learning and personal growth has been truly inspiring. Your willingness to face the difficult challenges it included with patience and persistence has been remarkable, and I am honored to have been a part of your journey.

As we approach the end of our journey together, I encourage you to take some time to reflect on all that we have learned and experienced. The wisdom we have gained together will serve as a valuable guide as you continue your journey toward a more fulfillings life. If you found this experience as life changing as it was for me then make sure to give it a positive review for those in doubt about reading it.

Remember to stay mindful, compassionate, and resilient in your daily life. Embrace each moment as an opportunity to learn and connect with yourself and those around you. The seeds we have sown together will continue to grow and bear fruit, and I am here to support you every step.

Thank you again for allowing me to be a part of your journey towards greater well-being and personal growth. Your commitment to self-improvement inspires us all, and I look forward to seeing all the amazing things you will achieve in the future.

With warm regards,
Gloria Clark

Made in United States
Troutdale, OR
06/05/2024

20341019R00055